The Habit Rollover Ultimate Fitness Planner

Mike Whitfield, Master CTT

The Habit Rollover

The Habit Rollover

HABIT ROLLOVER

Congratulations. You've already created momentum with your fitness journey by investing in this planner. Now you know you're serious ☺

During my journey of losing 115+lbs and keeping it off, I've discovered a very powerful method when it comes to losing weight. It's not a secret diet or pill, either (I think you've seen enough of that anyway).

Nope. This is so much more powerful. And it's worked for clients like Chris, who lost over 100lbs. It worked for Robin, a grandmother, who lost over 50lbs and 15% body fat. I can go on and on. It's so powerful, you can find yourself getting out of strongholds such as reaching into a bag of chips for the 10th time or stopping at Krispy Kreme on a Tuesday just because the "Hot Now" sign is on. ☺

So what is it?

The Habit Rollover

We'll first break it down and then you'll see how to create momentum using this method (and this planner) to get in the best shape of your life without feeling overwhelmed or deprived. Sound good?

Let's do this!

STEP 1: LIST YOUR TOP 4 HABITS

Habits come down to one of three categories:

1. A habit you need to implement
Example: Exercise 3 times a week

2. A habit you need to adjust
Example: Drink more water

3. A habit you need to remove
Example: Smoking

Don't overthink this. Just write down 4 habits you know fall into one the categories above. This is where customization comes into play.

For example – some people have no problem exercising but struggle with their food. Some people have no problem eating healthy food, but struggle to stay on a consistent exercise routine.

Write down the top four habits that come to mind. This will take anywhere between 5 to 15 minutes. Right now, it doesn't matter what order you put them in, either.

So now is the time to just jot down whatever comes to mind:

Habit 1: _____

Habit 2: _____

Habit 3: _____

Habit 4: _____

Next, we're going to create a game plan and it all starts by doing this...

STEP 2: WRITE WHAT YOU'RE CURRENTLY DOING VS WHAT YOU SHOULD BE DOING

Now let's create a game plan on mastering these habits.

For each habit, you'll want to write down what you're currently doing, and what you SHOULD be doing. Here's an example:

Habit #1: What I currently do:

NOT drink enough water

Habit #1: What I SHOULD do:

Drink 80oz of water a day

Habit #2: What I currently do:

Hit the gym 1-2 times a month

Habit #2: What I SHOULD do:

Exercise 3 days a week

Habit #3: What I currently do:

Eat a huge bowl of Lucky Charms every night

Habit #3: What I SHOULD do:

Enjoy some Greek yogurt or stop eating after dinner so I sleep better

Habit #4: What I currently do:

Never plan my meals so I end up eating fast food 4-6 times a week

Habit #4: What I SHOULD do:

Take some time on Sundays to plan my meals for the week

STEP 3: LIST YOUR HABITS IN ORDER FROM EASIEST TO HARDEST

Now that you have your habits in front of you (and what to do about them), list them in order from EASIEST to HARDEST to master.

Again, this comes down to customization (which is why this works so well). So, an example list might be something like this:

Easiest Habit:
Enjoy some Greek yogurt at night or stop eating after dinner

Second Easiest Habit:
Plan my meals on Sundays

Third Easiest Habit:
Exercise 3 times a week

Fourth Easiest Habit:
Drink 80oz of water every day

Your habits (and what you find easier) will be different and that's why this works (notice a "theme" here?) So let's list yours now:

Easiest Habit:

Second Easiest Habit:

Third Easiest Habit:

Fourth Easiest Habit:

Next up, you start attacking these habits one at a time...

STEP 4: YOUR WEEKLY PLAN TO DOMINATE YOUR HABITS

In your first week, you're going to attack habit 1 (easiest habit). **You go all in**. **Ignore all of the other habits.**

Your ultimate goal: Master this first habit for a minimum of 7 days straight. You DO NOT move onto the next habit until you've mastered your first habit.

Once you master your first habit, you "roll over" that habit into the following week while implementing habit #2.

For example:

Week 1: You nailed habit #1 5 out of 7 days.

Week 2: You nailed habit #1 7 days straight. Now you can "roll" that habit over while working on your next habit.

Week 3: You keep up habit #1 while implementing habit #2.

You get the idea.

You keep setting up these 4-week "blocks" using this habit-rollover approach.

Each week, you'll create more and more momentum. Next thing you know, your waistline is shrinking ☺ The idea is to NOT move onto the next habit until you've mastered the previous habit. For some habits, this will take a week. For others, it could take several weeks - even months. That's the idea. You want to master them so your weight loss efforts become "automatic" and not such a chore.

Now that you see how it works, let's get to work and leverage your planner. Want faster results? Leverage accountability.

Accountability is a powerful tool and it's not used enough. Accountability is a weapon against mass distraction, and it speeds up your success rate. When it comes to accountability, you either did or didn't do the thing you said you were going to do. That's where this journal can change your life. Want even better results from it? Connect with someone (or even start a group!) once a week and go over this journal with them.

Now if you don't have a specific goal for that day (for example – let's say your habit is to exercise 3 days a week - Monday, Wednesday, and Friday), feel free to circle "Yes" in your journal on a Tuesday. (Psychologically, it "preps" your mind to stick to it the following day, too ;)

By writing down your habit goals every day, this reinforces your "will" to stick to them. That's why the journal is designed this way.

Gear up. The next 12 weeks are going to be life changing!

My Habit Goal(s) This Week:

_____

_____

_____

_____

Did you stick to it?

Sunday: Yes   No

Reflection:

_____

_____

_____

_____

_____

_____

_____

_____

_____

My Habit Goal(s) This Week:

_____

_____

_____

_____

Did you stick to it?

Monday: Yes   No

Reflection:

_____

_____

_____

_____

_____

_____

_____

_____

_____

My Habit Goal(s) This Week:

_____

_____

_____

_____

Did you stick to it?

Tuesday: Yes   No

Reflection:

_____

_____

_____

_____

_____

_____

_____

_____

_____

My Habit Goal(s) This Week:

_____

_____

_____

_____

Did you stick to it?

Wednesday: Yes   No

Reflection:

_____

_____

_____

_____

_____

_____

_____

_____

_____

My Habit Goal(s) This Week:

_____

_____

_____

_____

Did you stick to it?

Thursday: Yes   No

Reflection:

_____

_____

_____

_____

_____

_____

_____

_____

My Habit Goal(s) This Week:

_____

_____

_____

_____

Did you stick to it?

Friday: Yes   No

Reflection:

_____

_____

_____

_____

_____

_____

_____

_____

_____

My Habit Goal(s) This Week:

_____

_____

_____

_____

Did you stick to it?

Saturday: Yes   No

Reflection:

_____

_____

_____

_____

_____

_____

_____

_____

_____

My Habit Goal(s) This Week:

_____

_____

_____

_____

Did you stick to it?

Sunday: Yes   No

Reflection:

_____

_____

_____

_____

_____

_____

_____

_____

My Habit Goal(s) This Week:

_____

_____

_____

_____

Did you stick to it?

Monday: Yes   No

Reflection:

_____

_____

_____

_____

_____

_____

_____

_____

My Habit Goal(s) This Week:

_____

_____

_____

_____

Did you stick to it?

Tuesday: Yes   No

Reflection:

_____

_____

_____

_____

_____

_____

_____

_____

_____

My Habit Goal(s) This Week:

_____

_____

_____

_____

Did you stick to it?

Wednesday: Yes   No

Reflection:

_____

_____

_____

_____

_____

_____

_____

_____

_____

My Habit Goal(s) This Week:

_____

_____

_____

_____

Did you stick to it?

Thursday: Yes   No

Reflection:

_____

_____

_____

_____

_____

_____

_____

_____

_____

_____

My Habit Goal(s) This Week:

_____

_____

_____

_____

Did you stick to it?

Friday: Yes   No

Reflection:

_____

_____

_____

_____

_____

_____

_____

_____

_____

My Habit Goal(s) This Week:

_____

_____

_____

_____

Did you stick to it?

Saturday: Yes   No

Reflection:

_____

_____

_____

_____

_____

_____

_____

_____

_____

My Habit Goal(s) This Week:

_____

_____

_____

_____

Did you stick to it?

Sunday: Yes   No

Reflection:

_____

_____

_____

_____

_____

_____

_____

_____

My Habit Goal(s) This Week:

_____

_____

_____

_____

Did you stick to it?

Monday: Yes   No

Reflection:

_____

_____

_____

_____

_____

_____

_____

_____

_____

My Habit Goal(s) This Week:

_____

_____

_____

_____

Did you stick to it?

Tuesday: Yes   No

Reflection:

_____

_____

_____

_____

_____

_____

_____

_____

My Habit Goal(s) This Week:

_____

_____

_____

_____

Did you stick to it?

Wednesday: Yes   No

Reflection:

_____

_____

_____

_____

_____

_____

_____

_____

_____

_____

My Habit Goal(s) This Week:

_____

_____

_____

_____

Did you stick to it?

Thursday: Yes   No

Reflection:

_____

_____

_____

_____

_____

_____

_____

_____

_____

My Habit Goal(s) This Week:

_____

_____

_____

_____

Did you stick to it?

Friday: Yes   No

Reflection:

_____

_____

_____

_____

_____

_____

_____

_____

_____

My Habit Goal(s) This Week:

_____

_____

_____

_____

Did you stick to it?

Saturday: Yes   No

Reflection:

_____

_____

_____

_____

_____

_____

_____

_____

_____

My Habit Goal(s) This Week:

_____

_____

_____

_____

Did you stick to it?

Sunday: Yes   No

Reflection:

_____

_____

_____

_____

_____

_____

_____

_____

My Habit Goal(s) This Week:

_____

_____

_____

_____

Did you stick to it?

Monday: Yes   No

Reflection:

_____

_____

_____

_____

_____

_____

_____

_____

My Habit Goal(s) This Week:

_____

_____

_____

_____

Did you stick to it?

Tuesday: Yes No

Reflection:

_____

_____

_____

_____

_____

_____

_____

_____

_____

My Habit Goal(s) This Week:

_____

_____

_____

_____

Did you stick to it?

Wednesday: Yes   No

Reflection:

_____

_____

_____

_____

_____

_____

_____

_____

_____

My Habit Goal(s) This Week:

_____

_____

_____

_____

Did you stick to it?

Thursday: Yes   No

Reflection:

_____

_____

_____

_____

_____

_____

_____

_____

_____

My Habit Goal(s) This Week:

_____

_____

_____

_____

Did you stick to it?

Friday: Yes   No

Reflection:

_____

_____

_____

_____

_____

_____

_____

_____

My Habit Goal(s) This Week:

_____

_____

_____

_____

Did you stick to it?

Saturday: Yes   No

Reflection:

_____

_____

_____

_____

_____

_____

_____

_____

My Habit Goal(s) This Week:

_____

_____

_____

_____

Did you stick to it?

Sunday: Yes   No

Reflection:

_____

_____

_____

_____

_____

_____

_____

_____

_____

My Habit Goal(s) This Week:

_____

_____

_____

_____

Did you stick to it?

Monday: Yes   No

Reflection:

_____

_____

_____

_____

_____

_____

_____

_____

_____

My Habit Goal(s) This Week:

_____

_____

_____

_____

Did you stick to it?

Tuesday: Yes   No

Reflection:

_____

_____

_____

_____

_____

_____

_____

_____

_____

My Habit Goal(s) This Week:

_____

_____

_____

_____

Did you st ck to it?

Wednesday: Yes   No

Reflection:

_____

_____

_____

_____

_____

_____

_____

_____

_____

My Habit Goal(s) This Week:

_____

_____

_____

_____

Did you stick to it?

Thursday: Yes   No

Reflection:

_____

_____

_____

_____

_____

_____

_____

_____

_____

My Habit Goal(s) This Week:

_____

_____

_____

_____

Did you stick to it?

Friday: Yes   No

Reflection:

_____

_____

_____

_____

_____

_____

_____

_____

_____

My Habit Goal(s) This Week:

_____

_____

_____

_____

Did you stick to it?

Saturday: Yes   No

Reflection:

_____

_____

_____

_____

_____

_____

_____

_____

_____

My Habit Goal(s) This Week:

_____

_____

_____

_____

Did you stick to it?

Sunday: Yes   No

Reflection:

_____

_____

_____

_____

_____

_____

_____

_____

My Habit Goal(s) This Week:

_____

_____

_____

_____

Did you stick to it?

Monday: Yes   No

Reflection:

_____

_____

_____

_____

_____

_____

_____

_____

My Habit Goal(s) This Week:

_____

_____

_____

_____

Did you stick to it?

Tuesday: Yes   No

Reflection:

_____

_____

_____

_____

_____

_____

_____

_____

_____

My Habit Goal(s) This Week:

_____

_____

_____

_____

Did you stick to it?

Wednesday: Yes   No

Reflection:

_____

_____

_____

_____

_____

_____

_____

_____

_____

My Habit Goal(s) This Week:

_____

_____

_____

_____

Did you stick to it?

Thursday: Yes   No

Reflection:

_____

_____

_____

_____

_____

_____

_____

_____

_____

My Habit Goal(s) This Week:

_____

_____

_____

_____

Did you stick to it?

Friday: Yes   No

Reflection:

_____

_____

_____

_____

_____

_____

_____

_____

_____

My Habit Goal(s) This Week:

_____

_____

_____

_____

Did you stick to it?

Saturday: Yes   No

Reflection:

_____

_____

_____

_____

_____

_____

_____

_____

_____

My Habit Goal(s) This Week:

_____

_____

_____

_____

Did you stick to it?

Sunday:　Yes　No

Reflection:

_____

_____

_____

_____

_____

_____

_____

_____

_____

My Habit Goal(s) This Week:

_____

_____

_____

_____

Did you stick to it?

Monday: Yes   No

Reflection:

_____

_____

_____

_____

_____

_____

_____

_____

My Habit Goal(s) This Week:

_____

_____

_____

_____

Did you stick to it?

Tuesday: Yes   No

Reflection:

_____

_____

_____

_____

_____

_____

_____

_____

My Habit Goal(s) This Week:

_____

_____

_____

_____

Did you stick to it?

Wednesday: Yes   No

Reflection:

_____

_____

_____

_____

_____

_____

_____

_____

My Habit Goal(s) This Week:

_____

_____

_____

_____

Did you stick to it?

Thursday: Yes   No

Reflection:

_____

_____

_____

_____

_____

_____

_____

_____

My Habit Goal(s) This Week:

_____

_____

_____

_____

Did you stick to it?

Friday: Yes   No

Reflection:

_____

_____

_____

_____

_____

_____

_____

_____

_____

My Habit Goal(s) This Week:

_____

_____

_____

_____

Did you stick to it?

Saturday: Yes   No

Reflection:

_____

_____

_____

_____

_____

_____

_____

_____

My Habit Goal(s) This Week:

_____

_____

_____

_____

Did you stick to it?

Sunday: Yes   No

Reflection:

_____

_____

_____

_____

_____

_____

_____

_____

_____

My Habit Goal(s) This Week:

_____

_____

_____

_____

Did you stick to it?

Monday: Yes   No

Reflection:

_____

_____

_____

_____

_____

_____

_____

_____

_____

My Habit Goal(s) This Week:

_____

_____

_____

_____

Did you stick to it?

Tuesday: Yes   No

Reflection:

_____

_____

_____

_____

_____

_____

_____

_____

_____

My Habit Goal(s) This Week:

_____

_____

_____

_____

Did you stick to it?

Wednesday: Yes   No

Reflection:

_____

_____

_____

_____

_____

_____

_____

_____

My Habit Goal(s) This Week:

_____

_____

_____

_____

Did you stick to it?

Thursday: Yes   No

Reflection:

_____

_____

_____

_____

_____

_____

_____

_____

_____

My Habit Goal(s) This Week:

_____

_____

_____

_____

Did you stick to it?

Friday: Yes   No

Reflection:

_____

_____

_____

_____

_____

_____

_____

_____

My Habit Goal(s) This Week:

_____

_____

_____

_____

Did you stick to it?

Saturday: Yes   No

Reflection:

_____

_____

_____

_____

_____

_____

_____

_____

My Habit Goal(s) This Week:

_____

_____

_____

_____

Did you stick to it?

Sunday: Yes   No

Reflection:

_____

_____

_____

_____

_____

_____

_____

_____

_____

My Habit Goal(s) This Week:

_____

_____

_____

_____

Did you stick to it?

Monday: Yes No

Reflection:

_____

_____

_____

_____

_____

_____

_____

_____

_____

My Habit Goal(s) This Week:

_____

_____

_____

_____

Did you stick to it?

Tuesday: Yes   No

Reflection:

_____

_____

_____

_____

_____

_____

_____

_____

My Habit Goal(s) This Week:

_____

_____

_____

_____

Did you stick to it?

Wednesday: Yes   No

Reflection:

_____

_____

_____

_____

_____

_____

_____

_____

_____

My Habit Goal(s) This Week:

_____

_____

_____

_____

Did you stick to it?

Thursday: Yes   No

Reflection:

_____

_____

_____

_____

_____

_____

_____

_____

_____

My Habit Goal(s) This Week:

_____

_____

_____

_____

Did you stick to it?

Friday: Yes   No

Reflection:

_____

_____

_____

_____

_____

_____

_____

_____

My Habit Goal(s) This Week:

_____

_____

_____

_____

Did you stick to it?

Saturday: Yes   No

Reflection:

_____

_____

_____

_____

_____

_____

_____

_____

_____

My Habit Goal(s) This Week:

_____

_____

_____

_____

Did you stick to it?

Sunday: Yes   No

Reflection:

_____

_____

_____

_____

_____

_____

_____

_____

_____

My Habit Goal(s) This Week:

_____

_____

_____

_____

Did you stick to it?

Monday: Yes   No

Reflection:

_____

_____

_____

_____

_____

_____

_____

_____

My Habit Goal(s) This Week:

_____

_____

_____

_____

Did you stick to it?

Tuesday: Yes   No

Reflection:

_____

_____

_____

_____

_____

_____

_____

_____

_____

My Habit Goal(s) This Week:

_____

_____

_____

_____

Did you stick to it?

Wednesday: Yes   No

Reflection:

_____

_____

_____

_____

_____

_____

_____

_____

_____

My Habit Goal(s) This Week:

_____

_____

_____

_____

Did you stick to it?

Thursday: Yes   No

Reflection:

_____

_____

_____

_____

_____

_____

_____

_____

My Habit Goal(s) This Week:

_____

_____

_____

_____

Did you stick to it?

Friday: Yes   No

Reflection:

_____

_____

_____

_____

_____

_____

_____

_____

_____

My Habit Goal(s) This Week:

_____

_____

_____

_____

Did you stick to it?

Saturday: Yes   No

Reflection:

_____

_____

_____

_____

_____

_____

_____

_____

My Habit Goal(s) This Week:

_____

_____

_____

_____

Did you stick to it?

Sunday: Yes   No

Reflection:

_____

_____

_____

_____

_____

_____

_____

_____

_____

My Habit Goal(s) This Week:

_____

_____

_____

_____

Did you stick to it?

Monday: Yes   No

Reflection:

_____

_____

_____

_____

_____

_____

_____

_____

My Habit Goal(s) This Week:

_____

_____

_____

_____

Did you stick to it?

Tuesday: Yes No

Reflection:

_____

_____

_____

_____

_____

_____

_____

_____

_____

My Habit Goal(s) This Week:

_____

_____

_____

_____

Did you stick to it?

Wednesday: Yes   No

Reflection:

_____

_____

_____

_____

_____

_____

_____

_____

_____

My Habit Goal(s) This Week:

_____

_____

_____

_____

Did you stick to it?

Thursday: Yes   No

Reflection:

_____

_____

_____

_____

_____

_____

_____

_____

_____

My Habit Goal(s) This Week:

_____

_____

_____

_____

Did you stick to it?

Friday: Yes   No

Reflection:

_____

_____

_____

_____

_____

_____

_____

_____

My Habit Goal(s) This Week:

_____

_____

_____

_____

Did you stick to it?

Saturday: Yes   No

Reflection:

_____

_____

_____

_____

_____

_____

_____

_____

_____

My Habit Goal(s) This Week:

_____

_____

_____

_____

Did you stick to it?

Sunday: Yes   No

Reflection:

_____

_____

_____

_____

_____

_____

_____

_____

My Habit Goal(s) This Week:

_____

_____

_____

_____

Did you stick to it?

Monday: Yes   No

Reflection:

_____

_____

_____

_____

_____

_____

_____

_____

_____

My Habit Goal(s) This Week:

_____

_____

_____

_____

Did you stick to it?

Tuesday: Yes   No

Reflection:

_____

_____

_____

_____

_____

_____

_____

_____

My Habit Goal(s) This Week:

_____

_____

_____

_____

Did you stick to it?

Wednesday: Yes   No

Reflection:

_____

_____

_____

_____

_____

_____

_____

_____

My Habit Goal(s) This Week:

_____

_____

_____

_____

Did you stick to it?

Thursday: Yes   No

Reflection:

_____

_____

_____

_____

_____

_____

_____

_____

_____

My Habit Goal(s) This Week:

_____

_____

_____

_____

Did you stick to it?

Friday: Yes   No

Reflection:

_____

_____

_____

_____

_____

_____

_____

_____

_____

My Habit Goal(s) This Week:

_____

_____

_____

_____

Did you stick to it?

Saturday: Yes   No

Reflection:

_____

_____

_____

_____

_____

_____

_____

_____

_____

ABOUT THE AUTHOR

Mike Whitfield is a Master CTT and has lost 115lbs and has kept it off for over a decade. He coached multiple transformation contest winners by shifting from fad diets and hardcore workouts to his "Habit Rollover" approach. You can get his powerful coaching program and his book, *Rise + Hustle* for FREE (while supplies last) at **www.RiseandHustleBook.com**

Made in the USA
Middletown, DE
04 December 2019

79985179R00056